*Revealing the Most Effective Diet for
Getting Slim and Young Today!*

Lose Up To 30 Lbs in 2 Weeks!

Dedicated to those searching for real solutions

to sustainable weight and balance.

Table of Contents

Part 1:

What is the NEW Miracle Diet?

Science behind these two ingredients that create magic when eaten together.

What celebrities would love to know to rebuild their bodies, beauty, and balanced youthful hormones guaranteed!

The power of transformation is in your grasp when you follow this easy plan.

Part 2:

Master this technique and you'll never have to diet again.

How this diet helps to undo the habit of mindless eating and tips for creating a foundation mindset for the future. How this diet shrinks your stomach size painlessly.

Your life is not the movies you watch; how to be the star of your own life.

Part 3:

Make calories work for you and never be hungry on this diet.

The catalysts for fat break down and elimination.

Making miracle water naturally; never be deficient in minerals again.

Part 1:

What is the NEW Miracle Diet?

Science behind these two ingredients that create magic when eaten together.

What celebrities would love to know to rebuild their bodies, beauty, and balanced youthful hormones guaranteed!

The power of transformation is in your grasp when you follow this easy plan.

This diet is referred to as a miracle diet not only because is a very fast form of fat loss, but it transforms the shape of the body to one that was never thought possible. What is put into the mouth has the biggest effect on body shape, texture, and ability. The problem comes down to what is the best thing to put into the mouth that will make the greatest positive impact on the body and mind. This diet is the best anti-aging diet, revealing skin that you had as a young child, soft, supple, and dewy. Cheeks actually become rosy again as in youth. An innocence shines through that will make people stare and wonder what could make such a difference. There is an answer to this question which will be revealed. The mind becomes very calm and stable, and deep thought is aroused; it's as if time shows down and your aging slows down with it. With this awakening comes a hormonal balancing and leveling where there otherwise were deficiencies and lacks. The hormones start working at top levels and efficiency. The body goes into a continuous fat burning mode even while sleeping and it boosts the metabolism. In just 7 days on the diet, it is normal to lose 14 lbs and 30 lbs in 2 weeks. For those looking to lose the last 10-20 lbs, it is ideal; and for those needing to lose a lot more in a short amount of time then it's ideal.

There are only two ingredients in this diet, which makes it very easy and affordable, not to mention it has practically no down time to prepare and to take on the go. Eggs contain all essential amino acids, 13 vitamins and minerals including vitamin A, E, D, and K. Eggs *contain the highest value of protein and healthy fats, which keep you satiated longer. Just having eggs for breakfast will lower your calorie intake for the next 36 hours! Riboflavin, vitamin B12, B6, B5, iron, selenium, phosphorus, calcium, zinc, and folate are also high in eggs. One egg contains approx. 75 calories, 7 grams of protein, 5 grams of fat, and 1.6 grams of saturated fat. Proteins are the main building blocks of the body and are used to make all kinds of tissues and molecules for all structural and functional purposes. The body is able to utilize the protein in eggs, which contain all of the essential amino acids in the right ratios. Eggs can be said to be a perfect food because they contain in themselves almost all the nutrients we need, so this diet is not lacking in nutritional variety as some might* suggest. Eggs contain omega 3 fatty acids which are essential for healthy brain, heart, and bowel functioning. Eggs are among the best sources of choline, which is essential to proper brain functioning and signaling, such as in memory. Choline is extremely beneficial for pregnant and lactating women because it increases the child's immunity to stress-related illnesses and chronic issues. Increased amounts of choline changed the gene expressions for releasing cortisol, which is a hormone related with stress and metabolic disorders. Eating eggs will not only benefit a baby, but it will decrease the stress levels in the body. Choline is vitally essential against birth defects; fetuses require six to seven times more than adults. Lutein and zeaxanthin are antioxidants very beneficial for sustaining eye health and warding off degenerative eye diseases. If possible it is best to get free-range eggs because they are much more nutritious and contain more omega 3 fatty acids. Omega 3 enriched eggs are very beneficial in reducing triglycerides levels in the blood. If the ones at the supermarket are too expensive, try finding a local farmer who would be willing to provide you with some eggs. The cholesterol in eggs has caused many people to stop eating eggs, but one must understand that there are two kinds of cholesterol. Dietary (HDL) cholesterol is the fat-like substance found in eggs, eggs only have 1.5g of this kind of cholesterol. This kind of cholesterol doesn't really affect the amount of cholesterol circulating in the bloodstream. The kind of cholesterol that affects the amount in the bloodstream is certain saturated and

Trans fats. Eggs contain 212mg, but this cholesterol is important in the body. Cholesterol is essential to all cell membranes, brain functioning, immune system, women's health, and it is actually used to make hormones in our bodies! This is amazing if the hormone levels in the body are low and off balance. LDL cholesterol is the 'bad' kind of cholesterol because it coats the blood vessels with this cholesterol and fat. What's amazing is that HDL cholesterol found in eggs will remove the LDL cholesterol from the blood vessels. That is why heart patients are medically inclined to eat a diet high in eggs. The 'good' cholesterol balances out the 'bad' cholesterol.

Oranges are the second ingredient in this diet. Oranges contain 93% vitamin C, fiber, folate, vitamin

B1, pantothenic acid, copper, potassium, and calcium. Oranges contain flavonoids which, lower high blood pressure and inflammation (asthma, osteoarthritis, and rheumatoid arthritis). These flavonoids are found in the peel and inner white pulp surrounding the oranges, so please make sure to eat the white pulp as well. The vitamin C in oranges prevents cholesterol from building up and sticking to the artery walls. Oranges are great for immune protection and provide the most significant protection against cancer, along with other citrus fruits. An orange has 170 different phytonutrients and more than 60 flavonoids, which are beneficial for eliminating inflammation, cancer, and blood clots. The polyphenols so abundant in oranges provide major antioxidant benefits for the whole body system. An active compound in oranges is called limonene and it lowers the 'bad' cholesterol in the body, which coupled with eggs is an amazing combination against heart and stroke disease. In addition to this, orange peels contain a specific kind of flavonoids (PMFs) that lower cholesterol levels better than some prescription drugs without side effects. This diet is extremely beneficial for those suffering from high LDL cholesterol levels risking heart disease. Oranges contain fiber which will definitely counteract any constipation associated with this diet as well as reducing high cholesterol levels, balancing blood sugars levels, and providing protection for the colon. Another benefit of oranges is that they help to dissolve the calcium stones in kidneys, protect against stomach ulcers, respiratory ailments, arthritis, and cardiovascular ailments. The vitamin C in oranges is a good mood enhancer; people suffering from depression and chronic fatigue are vitamin C deficient. Together with the hormone enhancing and balancing effect of eggs and mood-elevating effect of oranges you will definitely feel the difference. Today we find celebrity figures taking advantage of vitamin C intravenously. It is believed that because 100% of the vitamin C is being delivered directly into the blood, it becomes 100% bioavailable to the body, but that isn't necessarily true. The IV does deliver 100% of the vitamin C into the blood, but what about the cells where free radicals, pathogens, toxins reside? The body requires proteins to transport the vitamin C into the cell and these proteins require sodium, as well as there often are not enough of these *proteins and open portals for the vitamin C to become 100% available to the cell. What happens is it circulates in the blood and is eventually just peed out. What is so revolutionary about this diet combination is that 100% of the vitamin C is absorbed together with the perfectly-bioavailable proteins from eggs, resulting in complete cell renewal. You will notice this miraculous change on the inside and outside of your body. So it is not the amount of expensive vitamin C that in injected into your bloodstream directly that makes the change, it is the amount of vitamin C that is delivered into the cell that makes the lasting change, and oranges have more than enough vitamin C to make a huge difference in your youth and health.*

This diet plan has a few rules, but it is very easy to follow and sustain. First thing that needs to be mentioned is water. It is important to drink enough water because it will become a safeguard against cravings and losing control. When you drink 64 oz. of water first thing in the morning, it keeps you from having false cravings and binges. Adequate hydration will keep you feeling less hungry throughout the day. The water will be helping to eliminate toxins that will be rapidly releasing from your cells. It will keep you from being constipated throughout the day. With this diet it is usual to have a couple bowel movements per day. Drink 64 oz. of water first thing in the morning. The diet consists of 3 meals per day. Each meal is the same. Women eat two boiled eggs and one orange per meal. Men eat three boiled eggs and two oranges per meal. If you believe that you are not able to just jump into eating a small meal like this (for women), it is ok to start off with three boiled eggs and two oranges per meal for the first one to three days until you get used to it and are able to go down to two boiled eggs and one orange per meal. You will be able to reduce to smaller portions as the days go by because you will noticeably feel less and less hungry. Eggs are very satisfying on the satiation scale. Just eating an egg breakfast will keep a person eating fewer calories for the next 36 hours! **Rule # 1: Eat every 3-4 hours and DO NOT skip a meal!** If you skip a meal this will slow down your body's fat burning mode and your metabolism. Like a fire, just when it is still burning with embers and the room feels so warm, you have to put new logs into the embers because this will keep the temperature stable. If you skip you are more likely to binge. If you are having trouble waiting every 3 hours to eat, tell yourself things like its only one more hour I can wait...etc. **Rule # 2: The eggs must be boiling for 13 minutes!** This will keep you full, longer. **Rule # 3: Each bite you take, chew, chew, chew, at least 100 times per bite!** All these rules make for successful results and they must be adhered to. This may seem like a lot of times, but we need to stress the importance of chewing into your new eating habits. Digestion starts in the mouth not in the stomach. If you gulp down everything in 5 minutes it's not going to do its job of fat metabolism effectively. Another benefit for chewing 100 times per bite is that it teaches you to savor your food, be grateful for it, sense the subtle feeling of satiation and fullness, and most of all you will not feel as hungry in the following hours. The food should be liquefied completely before swallowing and bland of flavors or textures. Do not drink anything with your meal. If you are concerned about acid reflux, don't be, chewing enough times ensures proper food combination. **Rule # 4: Have a glass of water or decaf no- sugar tea two hours after your meal.** It's a good idea to wear a watch if you don't already or jot down your times on a notepad. After two hours from your meal, drink water or decaf herbal tea. Then an hour or two after you may have another meal. Do not eat two to three hours before bed. Before bed take a full spectrum trace mineral supplement. Minerals are very important for fat *metabolism, detoxification, and elimination. Your body is going through a lot of changes and it needs lots of time to do its job, so get at least 8 hours of sleep. Sleep is essential for maintaining balance in the body, fat metabolism, and when you get enough sleep you are less likely to overeat and crave unhealthy foods.*

Part 2:

Master this technique and you'll never have to diet

again.

How this diet helps to undo the habit of mindless eating

and tips for creating a foundation mindset for the future.

How this diet shrinks your stomach size painlessly.

Your life is not the movies you watch; how to be the star

of your own life.

All the rules that you adhere to is helping to build a proper foundation for your future eating habits. It takes 21-30 days to break a habit. If you can keep the rules for about a month, specifically one rule is most important and that it chewing 100 times per bite. Of course it depends how big your bites are, but you will learn to recognize when the food is really digested in the mouth as you do this longer, it will be completely liquefied and void of flavors. As this becomes second nature to you, it will be easy to recognize when the food is properly digested in your mouth instead of always counting up to 100 in your head. And as you start to eat different textured foods later on in your diet, you will recognize when the food is properly digested in your mouth and thus know when to swallow. Food becomes much more satisfying. If you feel awkward chewing that long then just take half the bite size and chew 50 times instead. When you follow this rule you will notice you will be full faster and you will sense satiation sooner, which will ensure not overeating. The reason for this is the more you chew the more energy is able to be converted out of your food because more enzymes are released in your mouth when you chew longer. When you chew more, the food entering into your stomach will be able to be broken down even further by the gastric juices, and when it enters into your small and large intestine all the nutrients will be fully absorbed. When this becomes a habit, you will eventually be able to eat anything you desire because you will be in tune to your bodies signals of satiation and you will know when to stop before over consuming calories. If you are not sure or not ready to make this commitment today then try this next time you eat: **Take small bites and chew 30 (least) -50 times per bite, (you will be delightfully surprised how much more satisfying and delicious the food is) and when you notice your body taking in its first breath or 'stomach' inhale, stop eating. It's that simple.** You will begin to notice a change instantly. Your first deeper than usual breath (usually from your stomach area) is what's meant as your 'stomach' inhale, everyone experiences this, but they ignore it and keep eating when their stomach is actually telling them that *"it's time to stop eating now, I'm full."* Even if you do not go on this diet, but just follow this rule all the time you will lose weight and feel much better. It's still wise to incorporate an eggs breakfast every day or an eggs meal every day because they are very nutritious and satisfying. Also opt out for more fresh produce and natural foods in your diet.

Mindful eating is very important on this diet. Focusing on your food during meal times will help you get through much more easily. Eating at a table is important because you want to see the food close in front of you. Chewing food is the key because it allows your taste buds to sense the flavors and textures more fully and longer. This will make satiation come sooner. Enjoy every bite, savor every flavor and texture, and chew until there are no more flavors left, 100 times per bite. Turn off all noise and avoid distractions during your meal time to really take in the meal time. Don't *look at the television or read a magazine or book, which is unconscious eating. Your attention needs to be focused on what's in front of you. If you do not do this you will be hungry sooner and you may feel like you're being deprived as if you haven't eaten at all. It's about training your senses; it takes effort at first, but the more you do it the more natural it will become and it won't be such an effort in the future. The first few days will be the hardest as you get used to the regime and if you are a dieter than you are most likely under nourished as you are not able to eat what your body desires because of calorie content etc… The limited quantity of food will be uncomfortable on your stomach as it will be shrinking to normal size. After the first couple days as your body adjusts and becomes re-nutritionalized, an awkward feeling starts to take place when you become less and less hungry but feel fuller. For a dieter who always feels hungry this is a very weird sensation, keep in mind your calorie content is fairly low even though you feel full to a point you don't want to eat anymore. This is all to do to the nutritional power-house in eggs. This small meal will become very satisfying and therefore your stomach will be shrinking back to its normal size very quickly. As your stomach will be contracting back to its normal size so will your waist and body. The more we eat, the more the stomach has to expand to accommodate that amount and then the more the body gains weight, it's all in the proportion of the stomach. Remember the stomach is the size of your fist or open palm, so imagine two eggs and an orange in your fist, they actually fit very snug. The* size of your fist is how much food you actually need to be eating in one sitting. Keep that in the back of your mind. The problem is that when we don't chew enough, we don't give the brain the time it needs (20 minutes) to send those 'full' feelings and before we know it we've eaten too much. Another reason is that the foods we eat are not naturally derived or nutritious enough to send those signals. Eating natural whole foods derived from the earth is what our bodies need. When we begin to eat mindfully, all those things we were using to ignore the problem of overeating will not be valuable as they were before. Wasting time watching how interesting other people's lives are will not be so thrilling anymore. Once you start to address your problem, you become the focus of your own life, not the lives of those on television. You are using television as a cover-up for all the things you wish you were and all the things you wish you could do. Stop ignoring your situation because now you have the answer on how to fix it. As you give more attention to working on that problem, your focus will naturally shift from the television back to yourself. Your life will become more interesting as you will have more energy, enthusiasm, and time to do those things that you want to do and to be the person you see yourself being. Give your personality and character a chance come out through your interests and in what makes you happy.

Part 3:

Make calories work for you and never be hungry on this diet.

The catalysts for fat break down and elimination.

Making miracle water naturally; never be deficient in minerals again.

We all know about calories, right? Well, it's not just about how many calories you eat, it's about the type of calories you eat. An egg contains approximately 75 calories but then so does a piece of chocolate. Which one will satisfy your bodies nutritional needs more? So you can agree that it really isn't about calories, it's about the type of food we eat that's important. Calories do and don't make a difference on this diet. Let me explain. When you are eating two eggs and a large orange, three times a day, you will be consuming just less than 700 calories a day. Your body will be burning excess fat stores as additional energy because these foods increase your metabolism to a point where you won't feel hungry. If you are a taller person and you require more calories, you might decide to eat three eggs and two oranges, three times a day, and then you will be consuming approximately 1,150 calories. Your body will also be burning excess fat stores as energy because these foods raise your metabolism as well. The more you eat the higher your metabolism will be, it has to be higher in order to burn those extra calories, even if you are overweight. If you are overweight and want to lose fat faster, than eat fewer calories on this diet to give your body the chance to burn more stored fat. It works on this diet because eggs satisfy your bodies hunger and are nutritionally dense, they rev up the metabolism, and coupled with oranges it creates a great fat-burning combination. As was mentioned earlier, you may want to start off having three eggs and two oranges per meal if you feel your will power is not 100%. As you progress *you will see that your appetite will go towards the smaller meals and you will lose weight faster.*

Minerals create biological balance, they are essential for all of the functions of the body, fat metabolism. This diet offers biologically available protein, that mean the body will be rebuilding itself rapidly and minerals are an essential element needed in building bones and teeth, skin, blood, hair, nerve function, muscle and metabolic processes. Minerals are needed to convert food into energy and vice versa, to turn stored energy (fat) back into usable energy. Minerals are needed for nutrient absorption and digestion. On this diet the body will be changing very rapidly so it is important to give it what it needs to do the job easily and without posing additional stress on the body. Minerals help to create that mental balance that we all need, especially on a diet. Minerals are meant to help you get through those challenges and mental lows that come with any change.

Bonus Secret Formula: How to create pure distilled living water.

#1 Truth: Nutrition means process of light energy.

Pour distilled water in a large glass jar and leave out in direct sunlight for 15 minutes. The water will ionize all known minerals like calcium, magnesium, and iron from the sunlight. These are bioavailable minerals (not rock powder) for our body. You will never have a mineral deficiency in your body again if you drink this miracle *water and incorporate natural sea salt (Celtic or*

Himalayan) into your diet.

www.ingramcontent.com/pod-product-compliance
Lightning Source LLC
Chambersburg PA
CBHW061936280526
45787CB00004B/1625